MEDICAL ETHICS: Real-World Application

Afshin Nasseri, MD

133 Clarendon St #170360, SMB 8584

Boston, MA 02117

Dedication

I would like to dedicate this book to, and thank my supportive wife, Seema, my beautiful and intelligent daughters Nazeela and Afshan, my parents, and my late in-laws, for their loving support.

Finally, I like to thank a great friend, Joseph Mazza, MD for his support and mentorship, throughout my professional life.

"a license to practice medicine is not an entitlement. License to practice medicine is only a privilege which physicians are trusted with and should always treasure and protect"

About,

Afshin Nasseri, MD, ACP

Dr. Nasseri has dedicated most of his adult life to internal medicine with interests in areas of geriatric medicine and noninvasive aesthetic medicine. He is an accomplished member of the American College of physicians and the Harvard's Institute of coaching, American Society of laser medicine and American bariatric physician Society. He is a member of Mindful Based Stress Reduction (MBSR) at Brown University.

He has been an accredited teacher to Brown and Boston University medical students and interns.

Dr. Nasseri is an active member of Grace Cares NGO, extending healthcare and education to remote and underprivileged areas. Through collaboration with a variety of organizations he has also funded a free medication program in these remote areas.

My personal experience

A few years ago, I underwent a stressful period in my professional life with many external factors contributing to the cause of my stress.

I ultimately learned that I am the one to be blamed the most. I failed to structure a good work and life balance framework the way I should have.

Learning the first lesson of self-accountability, led me to my pursuit of coaching and directing self-realization.

I am a member of the Harvard Institute of coaching and Brown University Center for Mindfulness, as a certified Health and Wellness and Leadership Coach.

Why I became a coach

The growing demands on Physicians and patients in the Healthcare industry, has taken its toll on traditional physician and patient relationship. Doctors are questioned about their recommendations as patients have become overnight doctors by their medical education on the internet. This evolution has led to dissatisfaction in a once respected and valued relationship. Private insurance companies have also done their part by undermining physicians' authority.

Physicians are retiring at a younger age or redirect their talents to other non- clinical professions. Patients must wait in line to find a primary care physician, or specialist alike.

Consumerism has become a behavioral norm, which has further strained the physician-patient relationship.

Physicians, and patients, as a part of a global population are all facing burnout. Anxiety and depression are noted at an alarming growth.

I hope that through Mindfulness, and self-realization I can redirect our focus, and make mindful decisions to enjoy the gift of "Life".

Preface

My name is Afshin Nasseri, and I have been practicing Internal Medicine for over twenty years. My formal training was completed at Brown University and Boston University, and I am presently an active member of the Harvard Institute of Coaching.

You may have acquired this book as a result of your experience with peers, administrators, patients, or State Medical Boards, where the outcomes of those interactions, have left you wondering, "…what if I had done things differently?"

In that case, I hope that this book answers some of your questions and guides you in future quandaries you may encounter.

If you are a healthcare worker seeking to understand the subject of medical ethics, then I hope that, this book helps you acquire the clarity you seek.

If you are an individual simply curious about medical ethics, then I raise my hat to you for your pursuit of knowledge.

Please ensure that you review the test questions included within this book, as they simulate real challenges in clinical practice.

CHAPTER 1

One of the most important steps in becoming a doctor is to take the Hippocratic oath, a promise to "first, do no harm." As a matter of fact, the first "do no harm" is attributed to "Of the Epidemics" one of Hippocrates' works, stating, "...the physician must be able to tell the antecedents, know the present, and foretell the future; [the physician] must mediate these findings, and have two special objects in view with regard to disease, namely, to do good or to do no harm."

What is Medical Ethics?

For the sake of argument let us consider that matters of ethics appear to be innate, and not studied. This presumption is logical, as ethics and "do no wrong" are learned at home, from family, friends, and mentors. However, society and medical boards need to have guidelines to adhere to for justice to be served, and thus, to protect the public.

The subject matter, admittedly, is not the most exciting, and the content may appear basic or obvious. Keep in mind that everyone has a violation potential which can jeopardize his/her medical license. Presenting these cases in clinical settings will enhance a higher level of engagement and learning through reflection.

CHAPTER 2

CODE OF ETHICS AND PROFESSIONALISM

<u>Study of Medical Ethics</u>

Medical ethics are learned by observing experienced physicians' practices and actions. Ethics are learned at home and through the family, and not at medical institutions. The importance of ethics in medical education cannot be understated, yet sadly, the subject of ethics does not play a major role in the medical school curriculum.

Ethics have been one of the building blocks of medicine since the time of Hippocrates, where the medical profession was first conceptualized, and the first public promise was made for physicians to place the interests of the patients above their own.

The subject of Medical Ethics has evolved and been influenced by multiculturalism, the development of human rights, and governmental and administrative contributions. Medical ethics are also closely analyzed in parallel to the law, and medical licensing authorities

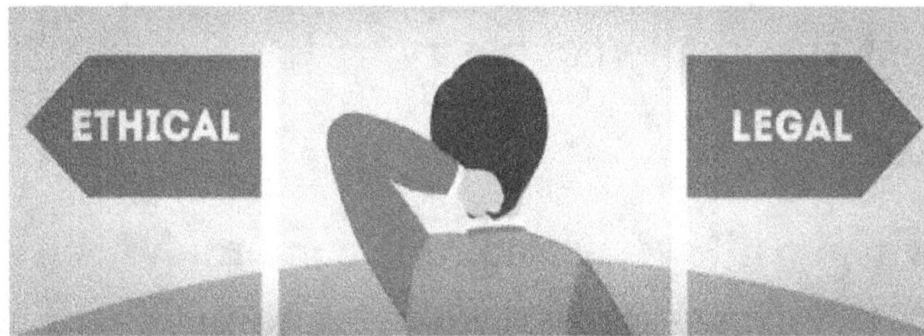

sanction physicians for ethics violations. Ethics mandate higher standards than the law, and where the law falls short, ethics is considered the prevailing factor in medical licensure adjudication.

The ethical physician is exemplified by virtues such as **compassion**, where the physician recognizes vulnerability and suffering, and attempts to understand each patient in order to alleviate the patient's condition.

The **Honest** physician is forthright and makes every attempt to communicate the truth - despite sensitivities - to the patient in a respectful manner.

Humility serves as a barrier for the physician to not overstep the limits of his/her knowledge and skills, or the limits of medicine, and encourages the physician to collaborate and seek support from colleagues when needed.

The physician with **integrity** consistently demonstrates his/her intentions through thought processes and actions by acting in a truthful manner in accordance with professional expectations, despite potential adversity.

The **prudent** physician uses his/her best clinical capabilities and moral reasoning to make thoughtful decisions in good conscience regarding medical care.

Being Honest

A physician must be forthright, respectful of the truth, and must both demand and communicate truth both sensitively and respectfully.

Code of Ethics

Do the right thing.

This sounds rather trivial and simple, but it is not. Opinions vary about every medical issue raised in private, public, and governmental forums. But which opinion is right?

Medical ethics set guidelines and principles to help us make decisions as physicians, however, these guidelines may come into conflict with each other. In such cases, options must be weighed via logic and ethical theories. Medical ethics explore subjective areas of decision-making, as decisions are usually not binary.

Consider the following cases:

1-Dr. You, is again faced with a patient with multiple comorbidities who makes a follow up appointment and as soon as her medications are called in to the pharmacy, she no-shows, or cancels the appointment and is nowhere to be found, no working phone, and mail returned.

2-Dr. Me becomes increasingly frustrated with patients or their family members who call after hours, particularly on Friday evenings and requesting pain killers for their older family members in pain, despite previous warnings.

3-Dr. Z is becoming increasingly frustrated with patients who come to him after consulting another health practitioner for the same illness. She considers this to be a waste of health resources and counter-productive for the health of the patients. She decides to tell these patients that she will no longer treat them if they continue to see other practitioners for the same condition.

4-Dr. X discovers that his patient of 15 years, is in violation of her pain management agreement and confronts her. The patient apologizes and pleads not to be discharged from the practice. Two weeks later she drops off a letter at the front desk addressed to Dr. X, pleading not to dismiss her and how she appreciates his services for the past 15 years. Dr. X declined to engage in correspondence as violating the pain management contract has obvious consequences. After 4 weeks, the said patient complained to the Board of Medicine that she was kissed by Dr. X.

5-Dr. N is seeing a known patient for a routine visit. He claims that he was ill ten days ago and had to call out from work for a week. Dr. N asked if he was seen by a Doctor during his illness. "No, I did not, but please give me a medical note or I will lose my job, I have been a good patient to you…"

6-Dr. C, a third-year surgical resident is annoyed by the behavior of the senior surgeon in the operating room. The surgeon uses techniques that prolong operative time and cause greater post-operative pain, and longer post-op recovery times. Additionally, he constantly makes inappropriate jokes and intimidates the surgical assistants.

7-Dr. K examines a female patient with severe facial eczema. Patient had already been seen at a local walk-in clinic where she was given a Medrol Pak 3 days prior by a nurse practitioner, without any improvement and now advancing to periorbital area. Given the patient's level of discomfort, patient agreed to an intramuscular steroid injection. In two days, patient's eczema had completely resolved. She complained to Board of Medicine about a small dimple at the site of her injection.

Each of these cases mandate ethical reflection. They raise questions about physician behavior and decision-making. It is not about how to treat pheochromocytomas, hypertension or diabetes, it is about reflection, responsibilities, values, morality and rights. Physicians face these kinds of questions every day and truly one cannot generalize scenarios. Such profound decisions must be entertained in minutes. There are no in-house attorneys, ethics committees and no board rooms, it's the physicians, the patients and the oath they took.

Ethical questions in medicine are not all equally challenging. Some are relatively easy to answer, mainly because there is a well-developed consensus on the right way to act in particular situations, for example, the physician should always ask for a patient's consent before a procedure.

Ethics is the study of morality, reflection and analysis of moral decisions and driven behavior.

<u>**Medical Ethics**</u>

The American Medical Association has written a "Code of Medical Ethics" for healthcare providers facing ethical questions in their careers, which consists of guidelines and opinions written by ethics scholars and physicians. The American College of Physicians has also published a similar, yet concise, handbook of ethical guidelines.

Medical ethics consists of four pillar-like principles as an elementary guide to the practice of medicine. Each individual case can be analyzed, and the decision-making process can be facilitated, using these principles.

The four principles of medical ethics:

Autonomy: This relates to a patient's independence or freedom. A competent adult has the right to make decisions about what happens to his/her body. This person must be capable of rational thought process and not be coerced into a decision. An adult can refuse medical care or treatment or accept treatment when his provider suggests it. That patient then lives with the consequences of his/her decision.

A physician cannot examine you, do blood work, perform a colonoscopy, or treat your ear infection without your consent.

The rights to autonomy and confidentiality is limited where there is potential harm to an innocent third party.

Patient autonomy gives you the right to make the wrong choice about your healthcare regime. Even if you are unable to make your health-care choices, the physician cannot simply make decisions on your behalf. This stands even if your choices would be harmful to you.

This is one of the most difficult things for a physician to understand and abide by. Doctors are trained to act in the best interest of their patients, but a patient's right to act against his/her own best interest comes first.

Beneficence: A physician must act in the best interests of the patient. Providers are required to be engaged in their patient's health and well-being. Beneficence means providers must be committed to helping their patients.

Nonmaleficence: Physicians must not harm a patient through carelessness, malice, hatred, vengeance. This principle is balanced with beneficence, in that any risks of a treatment or procedure for a patient must be outweighed by the benefits. Procedures or treatments always carry a risk of harm, but when the treatment is very risky, the benefit must be greater than the risk of not performing the procedure.

"Double effect" is a derivative of nonmaleficence. This doctrine states that if doing something morally good has a bad outcome, it's ethical to do it providing the effect was unintentional. This is true even if with the foresight that the outcome was probable.

Justice: The principle of justice states that there should be an element of fairness in all medical decisions that both burden and benefit patients, as well as equal distribution of scarce resources and new treatments. Additionally, it is necessary for medical practitioners to uphold applicable laws and legislation when making choices.

Conflict of Interest

A Physician must resolve all conflicts of interest in the best interest of the patient.

A Physician must make full, transparent, and timely disclosure of any conflict of interest.

Physicians must NOT:

1. Seek or accept any benefit for a referral, service or product provided by another Physician to a patient, other than for services provided by a partner, associate, employee or locum of the primary Physician.
2. Offer an inducement to another Medical professional conditional on providing a referral, service or product to a patient, whether medically appropriate or not.
3. Encourage another person to offer or accept an inducement conditional on providing a referral, service or product to a patient, whether such referral, service or product is medically appropriate.
4. Refer a patient to any facility or healthcare business in which the Physician has a direct or indirect financial interest. There should be no terms or conditions that require the Physician to make referrals to a facility or generate business for a facility

CHAPTER 3

Decision Making & Competence

Competency is a legal term and determination of competency ultimately lies with the judicial system. All adult patients are considered competent unless specifically proven otherwise in a court of law. Physicians, however, can determine whether a patient has the capacity to properly comprehend his/her medical condition through neurological examinations including testing memory, comprehension, reasoning, and judgment. Furthermore, laboratory studies can be used to determine any organic abnormalities to determine any underlying pathology which may affect a patient's capacity.

Q1 A 30-year-old man in a motor vehicle accident presents to the emergency department. After extended resuscitation efforts, he develops anoxia. Poor neurological prognosis, his inability to regain consciousness was determined. The patient has no advanced directive and his spouse claims that the patient said that he would not want to be kept alive if he could not interact with his family.

What is the next step in management?

A-risk management evaluation

B-patient's medical condition

C-patient's best interest

D-patient's previously expressed wishes

Q2 A 30-year-old female presents in her last trimester. Her obstetrician has recommended a C-section given the large size of the fetus in comparison to the patient's pelvis. Patient declines going through surgery despite her full understanding of the procedure due to associated pain. She is informed that fetus may not survive without the C-section. What is the most appropriate decision-making process?

A - psychiatric evaluation

B -obtained a court order perform the surgery

C-discuss this matter with the baby's father asked for consent to perform surgery

D- honor the patient's wishes

Q3 A72-year-old man is evaluated for colon cancer metastasized to liver. Chemotherapy is could extend the patient's life by 12 to 18 months. The patient has mild dementia which started 18 months ago, and his wife has now manages family finances and driving. A Mini–Mental State Examination reveals a score of 22. The risk and benefits of chemotherapy and alternative treatments are explained to the patient and his wife.

Which is the best way to determine chemotherapy treatment for this patient?

A- Ask the patient if he wants chemotherapy

B- Ask the patient if he wants chemotherapy now and ask him again later

C- Ask the patient to repeat the key benefits and risks of chemotherapy

D- Ask the patient why he does or does not want chemotherapy

E- Defer decision to the patient's wife

CHAPTER 4

Informed consent

Medical decision-making is ideal in a setting where patients are empowered to make informed decisions regarding their health by being provided with adequate information regarding their health with respect and acceptance.

Consent is Implied in an Emergency

- Patients have the right to decide on investigations and treatments (patient autonomy).
- Mentally competent patients have the right to refuse/withdraw consent for treatments.
- Consent must be voluntary and informed.
- Patients must have the capacity to give consent.
- The physician is required to provide pertinent, objective information that a "reasonable" patient would want or need to make an informed decision.
- Elements of informed consent are diagnosis, proposed treatment, rate of success, risks, alternative treatments, non-treatment consequences, and responses to all questions
- Consent must be documented in the medical record and is required for each procedure
- The patient's decision must be respected.

Q4 Joseph, a 20-year old, presents to the emergency department in excruciating knee pain. She fell on asphalt yesterday while playing soccer and scraped his knee. His knee is now extremely swollen and painful, and he cannot bend or bear weight. You explain to Joseph that he has a septic knee which must be aspirated, and explain the risks associated with the aspiration. You're not certain that he fully understands the information since he is in such severe pain and appears apprehensive and afraid.

A-begin aspirating the knee

B-Try and locate a family member

C-Reassess if patient is alert and orient to time, place and person

D- attempt to get a verbal consent

Q5 A 60-year-old man has a 2-month history of chest pain and fainting spells. You feel his symptoms require cardiac catheterization. The risks and potential benefits are explained to him and his likely prognosis without the intervention. He verbalizes understanding of all of this but refuses the intervention.

Can the patient legally refuse the said intervention?

A-Yes, as the patient is competent to make this decision, and the doctor has a duty to respect his wishes.

B-No, because the patient does not comprehend the severity of his condition.

C-No, because the patient has a life-threatening condition.

D-Yes, but the doctor has the duty to obtain a court order.

CHAPTER 5

<u>Confidentiality</u>

The term 'confidentiality' refers to the protection of sensitive information. Health care providers respect confidentiality by protecting personal health information to others who have no right to the information and by safeguarding patient information from those without authorization. Providers can violate this duty both intentionally and unintentionally. An unethical physician might intentionally breach confidentiality by selling information about a celebrity patient to a journalist. A nurse might inadvertently violate confidentiality by discussing a patient's condition with a co-worker in a public area where it may be overheard by other patients or visitors.

Most prominent federal regulations implemented under the Health Insurance Portability and Accountability Act of 1996 (HIPAA). The foundation for these regulations was a perceived threat to patient confidentiality posed by electronic transmission of medical records, the HIPAA privacy regulations require health care providers to protect the confidentiality of personal health information (PHI) recorded or transmitted in any form, including electronic, written, and oral communication. Under these regulations, providers must obtain the patient's written authorization to use or disclose PHI. There are, however, notable exceptions to this requirement; providers may use and disclose PHI without patient authorization for "treatment, payment, and health care operations" activities, and for twelve "national priority purposes," including public health and abuse and neglect reporting requirements, law enforcement purposes, and organ donation. Violations of HIPAA privacy regulations may subject health care providers to civil and criminal penalties.

According to the Medical Patients' Rights Act, a law passed by Congress in 1996, all patients have the right to have their personal privacy respected and their medical records handled with confidentiality. Test results, patient histories, and even the confirmation that the person is a patient, cannot be passed on to another person without the patient's consent. No information can be given over the telephone without the patient's permission. No patient records can be given to another person or physician without the patient's written permission, unless the court has subpoenaed it.

Sharing health information amongst physicians at the time of a referral is common practice. However, the patient must consent for his/her information to be transferred to another physician by signing a release form.

The AMA appeals to an implied duty to obey the law which may override the duty to protect patient confidentiality. Some jurisdictions require health care professionals to report certain personal health information, including diagnoses of serious communicable diseases, abuse or neglect of children or older adults, gunshot and knife wounds, and poisonings, and so on.

These laws require reporting to public health, social services, or law enforcement officers. Enforcing of these reporting practices reflects a social choice that protection of the public's health and prosecution of serious crimes should override patient confidentiality. Information takes variety of forms. A neurologist providing medical care for a patient with a newly diagnosed seizure disorder and the likelihood of harm to public as a motor vehicle operator. The neurologist may report his assessment to appropriate state agency to suspend the patient's driver's license. Other examples are notifying authorities of a psychiatric patient's intention to harm self or others. Informing the wife of a patient diagnosed with HIV is another difficult yet necessary act.

Q6 An 82-year-old female with multiple comorbidities is diagnosed with lung cancer. She declines surgery, chemotherapy, or radiation therapy. She states that she has lived a good life and is too old for interventions. She lives with her older daughter and she also has a son. She requests that her condition to remain confidential. You determine that she is mentally competent to make that decision. She signs a do-not-resuscitate order and advance directives stating that she does not want to be kept alive by artificial means.

Both the son and daughter call requesting information about their mother's medical condition.

Who would you discuss the patient's condition with?

A- Neither daughter nor son

B- Both daughter and son

C- The daughter

D- The son

CHAPTER 6

Medical Records, Error & Correction

Legally speaking, medical records are owned by a Physician or health-care institution, but the information contained within the medical record is the property of the patient. The patient has an absolute right to access the information contained in the medical record, which is covered by all the same rules of confidentiality as any other privileged medical information.

In the case of a chart error, the doctor should draw a line through the error, and initial next to the correction. Hence, anyone reading the chart would see the original content, and this ensures that medical errors are not being concealed.

Pages cannot be removed from medical charts, and "white out" cannot be used. If a Physician forgets to put a note in the chart documenting a patient's condition on a prior day, the note cannot be backdated, and must always reference the current date and time.

A Physician cannot release a medical record without the consent of the patient, and no one except those directly involved in the care of the patient has a right to access the record.

Patients cannot take sole possession of the physical medical record, but they have a right to access or copy the information, and a medical record cannot be withheld to force a patient to settle medical bills. The patient's right to his/her medical record information outweighs the physician's unpaid medical bills.

Q7 Your patient requested a copy of her records from the community hospital. Her request was declined, as she needs a specific reason to obtain her records. She sees you at your office and is requesting your guidance. What should you tell her?

A-Only a healthcare institution, insurance company or physician can access her medical records.

B-The hospital will provide her the medical records if a physician asks

C-She has every right to have a copy of her records.

D-Only the physician can obtain and review her records.

Q8 A 60-year-old female presents to the clinic complaining of feeling faint and dizzy for the past two weeks. Her past medical history is significant for diabetes mellitus type II, hypertension and osteoarthritis. She takes metformin, lisinopril and occasional nonsteroidal anti-inflammatory drugs to alleviate discomfort from her osteoarthritis discomfort. Her documented blood pressure at the office two weeks ago was normal and the plan clearly indicates to maintain the same medical regimen. However, there is also a note in the chart from a colleague to increase the dose of her antihypertensive medication.

During the office visit, her blood pressure is at 110/60 with significant orthostatic changes upon standing. What will be your best course of action?

A-explain that pharmacy made an error in dosage

B-apologize and explain that a colleague made a mistake in her chart and apparently her blood pressure medication dosage was increased.

C-Resume previous dose of her lisinopril without any further disclosure

D-report the error to the medical board

CHAPTER 7

Physician Patient Relationship

The physician-patient relationship is the core of practice of medicine and is a relationship of confidentiality and trust. The physician must honor this sacred relationship by acting in the patient's best interests. Acceptance of all patients without discrimination, including age, disability, gender identity, language, marital and family status, medical condition, ethnic origin or political affiliations, religions, sex, sexual orientation and socioeconomic status, is necessary.

Patients are the most important assets to a practice. Sometimes, physicians encounter difficult patients who make them and their medical staff feel upset and frustrated. In these situations, understanding the patient's psychology and motivation is key. Staff members should also be trained on how to manage such patients. Ultimately, the physician is responsible for identifying such patients and managing them appropriately. Patient management skills include listening, providing attentiveness, expressing empathy, asking questions, making eye contact and always ending a visit on a positive note.

The way a Physician handles difficult patients will define the quality of the patient experience. Not knowing how to deal with difficult patients may lead to low staff morale, low patient volume and a damaged reputation for a practice.

Regardless of how good the service is within a practice; it is just a matter of time before the first encounter with a difficult patient. It is inevitable and unavoidable. Typically, a difficult patient will want to consume a physician's time and focus only on his/her issue, frustrate the Physician and staff in the process, and furthermore haggle endlessly to receive more time or to acquire "freebies."

Keep the following point in mind when dealing with difficult patients: A Physician has the right to refuse patients for legitimate reasons.

Physicians should limit self-treatment or treating family members and close friends to emergencies, and when no other physician is available. It is part of a physician's duty to provide emergency medical care when appropriate to anyone who is in need.

Q9 A 24-year-old female friend sends you an email requesting your opinion on her medical condition. She decided to contact you after reviewing your online profile. She is not an established patient. She claims to have had lower back and abdominal pain with alternating constipation and diarrhea. She takes fiber and laxatives. She has done testing by her primary care physician and gastroenterologist, including an upper endoscopy and colonoscopy. She requests your recommendation for another test or treatment. What is the most appropriate next step in management?

A-Ignore the email.

B-Request her medical records before any recommendation.

C-Advise the patient to be evaluated for celiac disease.

D-Advise patient to call your office to establish care.

Disclosure of Harm

When a patient suffers harm that negatively affects the patient's health or quality of life, the responsible physician must ensure that the patient receives full disclosure of that information.

Disclosure of harm is considered a process that also addresses the patient's immediate and future medical needs, and the investigation of the circumstances that led to the patient suffering harm, and furthermore, steps to prevent recurrence of such harm.

Disclosure must occur whether the harm is a result of disease progression, a complication of care, or an adverse event.

Disability Certification

Patients may report having been ill for one week at home, not attending work, requesting your certification for their absence, despite your lack of involvement during their illness. There are less fortunate patients with chronic debilitating illnesses, where society allows physicians to justify their illness to obtain different types of support, whether financial or otherwise. Physicians must always act honestly and be able to support decisions based on facts.

Sexual Relationships between Physician and Patient

Sexual relationships between a physician and a current patient are never ethical and constitute a violation of boundaries with severe consequences. The physician/patient relationship must cease in such a case, and the patient must be transferred to another physician, to ascertain clear boundaries.

The American Medical Association and the ACP both state that it is unethical for a physician to become sexually involved with a current patient even if the patient initiates or consents to the relationship. A lack of equality between the parties; a patient in a vulnerable and dependent state, and the physician indiscretion with confidential information and not acting in the patient's best interest are the foundation for such ethics-based recommendations. There are sanctions against these relationships, ranging from criminal charges to sanctions by state licensing boards. Sexual contact or a romantic relationship between a physician and a former patient may also be unethical regardless of time elapsed since ending the professional relationship. Physicians should avoid such relationships with a family member or surrogate of a patient. A physician should always consult with a colleague or other professional prior to becoming sexually involved with a former patient.

It has been reported that 5% to 10% of psychiatrists have had sexual contact with a patient; the statistics remain unknown of practitioners in other specialties. Physicians aware of instances of sexual misconduct have an obligation to report them.

CHAPTER 8

<u>Terminating the Physician-Patient Relationship</u>

•   A physician who terminates a relationship with a patient must have reasonable grounds for discharging the patient from the medical practice and must document those reasons in the patient's chart.

•   A physician must not discharge a patient based on protected categories, including age, gender, marital status, medical condition, national or ethnic origin, physical or mental disability, political affiliation, race, religion, sexual orientation, or socioeconomic status. Furthermore, a patient cannot be discharged due to poor lifestyle choices, failing to keep appointments, or failing to pay outstanding fees, unless several notices have been given to patient and documented.

•   Refusal to follow medical advice, and repeated non-adherence despite reasonable attempts by the physician to address the non-compliance, are grounds to discharge a patient.

•   A physician must give advance written notice of intention to terminate care and provide a timeline to advise the patient of the reasons for termination. This written notice must include the following:

(a)   Ensured continuity of follow-up care for outstanding treatments and medical conditions prior to the termination date or facilitation of transfer of care to another physician

(b)   Provision for emergency services that would otherwise be unavailable to the patient after the termination date

(c)   Transfer of the patient's medical information in response to future requests by the patient or an authorized third party.

A physician may immediately discharge a patient if:

(d)   the patient is abusive or poses a safety risk to office staff, other patients, or the Physician

(e)   the patient fails to respect professional boundaries

(f)   the Physician is leaving the medical practice

Q-8 A 40-year-old man with a history of hip osteoarthritis was evaluated. Months ago, for an office treatment which included weight loss, NSAIDs and physical therapy were prescribed. He was also seen at two different urgent care facilities requesting stronger medication to alleviate pain. He did not keep his appointment with you. Patient was also not available by telephone and his past medical history is significant for depressive disorder yet during his last office visit he did not appear suicidal or homicidal. What is the next step in management?

A-dispatch mental health crisis

B-terminate physician-patient relationship

C- send a formal letter to patient indicating that he may be discharged from the practice

D-refer the patient to a psychiatrist

CHAPTER 9

Medical Etiquette, Doctor to Doctor

There are certain standards of professional behavior, that physician's practice in their relationship and conduct other physicians. These behaviors are not considered to be medical ethics issues. A physician expects his/her phone calls to a fellow physician be taken promptly and be seen equally promptly when visiting a physician's office. This extension of courtesy exists since physicians are often consulting about patients with other physicians.

Ethical issues arise when one physician overlooks the medical deficiencies of another physician.

Q-11 A third-year surgical resident is concerned with the conduct of the senior surgeon in the operating room. The surgeon uses lengthy and outdated techniques resulting in greater post-operative pain and extended recovery times. He makes inappropriate jokes about the patients that which bothers and intimidates the nurses. Given the level of hierarchy, the resident is reluctant to discuss the matter with the surgeon or relay his conduct to higher authorities. But he feels that he must somehow improve the situation for all involved parties.

A-The resident has an ethical duty to disclose the unethical behavior, however he is still a physician in training, and he should discuss this with a senior physician.

B-The resident must have a discussion with the senior surgeon, if not successful, he should then report his behavior to the hospital administrators.

C-The resident should appoint the anesthesiologist to report the surgeon.

D-The anesthesiologist should appoint an assisting nurse to discuss the case with senior surgeon.

CHAPTER 10

Mental Health

A patient with the clear capacity to understand, or one who clearly does not have capacity, does not need a psychiatric evaluation. However, a mental health evaluation can help in questionable cases to further assess capacity. For example, suicidal patients lack the capacity to understand as active suicidal ideation is a sign of impaired judgment. Or, a patient may have a history of bipolar disorder making it impossible for him/her to manage his financial decisions.

However, the same individual might still be considered to have the competence to refuse treatment.

Most patients seen in primary care will experience one or more psychological or behavioral health problems during their lifetime. Although some patients need specialized care, primary care physicians should not discount the potential impact of taking time during office visits to consider brief behavioral interventions with patients who struggle emotionally or face life crises. Actions such as instilling hope, and using active listening can be powerful.

Physicians can also greatly influence patient willingness to follow through with referrals. With mental illness, however, the limits of primary care physicians' roles are less clear. What is correct in the case that a patient is hearing voices or walks into the office and announces that he/she has decided to kill him/herself? What about a lawyer who's having trouble meeting deadlines and asks for medication for attention-deficit disorder? Or the patient whose therapist told her to see her PCP about prescribing an antidepressant? Or the police officer who, after a shoulder injury, is trying to shake an Oxycontin addiction? The request for treatment in these cases is primarily due to a level of comfort with primary care physicians and lack of access to a psychiatrist.

Over a third of all mental-health care in the U.S. is now provided by primary-care doctors, nurse practitioners, pediatricians, and family practitioners, often because there are not enough practicing psychiatrists, thus, this burden falls on primary caregivers.

CHAPTER 11

Genetic Testing, Precision Medicine, Research

Precision medicine encompasses disease treatment, prevention, and risk stratification that considers individual genetic variations. This personalized approach includes:

1. Predictive genome testing done in asymptomatic individuals to determine whether an individual is at increased risk for disease
2. Diagnostic testing done to rule out or confirm a genetic condition, based on clinical characteristics in an affected individual
3. Pharmacogenomics for more focused prescribing
4. Molecular recognition of tumors to enhance therapy
5. Whole-genome sequencing to determine an entire genome for genetic mutations.

Precision medicine is not flawless, and raises several issues, such as patient and physician education, counseling, privacy, confidentiality, cost, patient's best interests, and legal matters.

Genomic testing may predict diseases and susceptibility without the ability to improve therapeutic measures for prevention or cure. Patients should be educated about the benefits, risks, limitations, and outcomes of genomic testing. A referral of the patient to a clinical geneticist or genetic counselor is the most prudent path given that physicians are not all regularly trained and educated on this subject matter.

Risks, benefits, limitations, and cost of testing must also be discussed with patients prior to testing. Unravelling data about uncertain or incidental findings could be detrimental to patients and their families by causing anxiety or a negative impact on well-being. Furthermore, the labeling or misuse of information by employers, insurers, or other institutions should be fully understood by the patient.

Many state and federal governments are enforcing rules on access by employers and insurers to genomic information. The Genetic Information Nondiscrimination Act of 2008 was designed to prevent discrimination in health insurance and employment based on genetic data. Patients should be well-informed about testing and disclosure of genetic information.

Q-12 The patient has a strong family history of breast cancer. She requests to perform BRCA genetic test to see if she has an increased risk for breast cancer. The patient's employer is requesting a copy of any genetic testing done on this patient.

A-provide information only if the result is positive

B-refuse to provide information

C-discuss the matter with your attorney

D-provide the employer with requested information.

RESEARCH IN MEDICAL PRACTICE

Medicine is not an exact science as in physics and math. Every patient is different and what may be an effective treatment for most of the population, may have side effects for the rest. Even the most widely accepted treatments must be monitored and evaluated to establish safety and efficacy.

All physicians make use of the results of medical research in their clinical practice. To maintain their competence, physicians must keep up with the current research in their area of practice through Continuing Medical Education. Even if they do not engage in research themselves, physicians must know how to interpret the results of research and apply them in in practice. A familiarity with research methods is essential for competent medical practice.

The most common path of research for practicing physicians is the clinical trial. Before a new drug can be approved by governmental agencies it must undergo extensive testing for safety and efficacy. Laboratory studies followed by testing on animals, if proven promising then the four phases of clinical research, follow:

- Phase one research, usually conducted on a relatively small number of healthy volunteers, who are often paid for their participation, is intended to determine what dosage of the drug is required to produce a response in the human body, how the body processes the drug, and whether the drug produces toxic or harmful effects.

- Phase two research is conducted on a group of patients who have the disease that the drug is intended to treat. Its goals are to determine whether the drug has any beneficial effect on the disease and has any harmful side effects.

- Phase three research is the clinical trial, in which the drug is administered to many patients and compared to another drug, if there is one for the condition in question, and/or to a placebo. Where possible, such trials are 'double-blinded', i.e., neither research subjects nor their physicians know who is receiving which drug or placebo.

- Phase four research takes place after the drug is licensed and marketed. For the first few years, a new drug is monitored for side effects that did not show up in the earlier phases. Additionally, the pharmaceutical company is usually interested in how well the drug is being received by physicians who prescribe it and patients who take it.

- PRINCIPLE ONE: Minimizing the risk of harm

- PRINCIPLE TWO: Obtaining informed consent

- PRINCIPLE THREE: Protecting anonymity and confidentiality

- PRINCIPLE FOUR: Avoiding deceptive practices

- PRINCIPLE FIVE: Providing the right to withdraw

The significant number of ongoing trials required seeking and enrolling larger numbers of patients to meet the statistical demands of the trials. Those in charge of the trials now rely on many more physicians, often in different countries, to enroll patients as research subjects.

Medical research is a well-funded enterprise, and physicians are sometimes offered considerable rewards for participating. These can include cash payments for enrolling research subjects, equipment such as computers to transmit the research data, invitations to conferences to discuss the research findings, and co-authorship of publications on the results of the research. The physician's interest in obtaining these benefits can sometimes conflict with the duty to provide the patient with the best available treatment. It can also conflict with the right of the patient.

The ethical values of the physician – compassion, competence, autonomy – apply to the medical researcher as well. So, there is no inherent conflict between the two roles. If physicians understand and follow the basic rules of research ethics, they should have no difficulty participating in research as an integral component of their clinical practice.

Social Value

One of the more controversial requirements of a medical research project is its contribution to the well-being of society in general. It used to be widely agreed that advances in scientific knowledge were valuable in themselves and needed no further justification. However, social value is an important criterion for approval of a project.

Informed Consent, the form being signed must involve a thorough oral explanation of the project and what it will mean to the research subject. Research subjects should be informed about freedom to withdraw their consent to participate at any time.

Q-13 A family practitioner in a rural town, is approached by a contract research organization to participate in a clinical trial of a new non-steroidal inhaler for asthma maintenance treatment. She is offered an amount of money for each patient that she recruits for the trial.

The C.R.O. representative assures her that all approvals have been obtained. Dr. has never participated in a trial and is eager to start. What should have been the appropriate action?

A-The doctor should not have accepted without ensuring that all the requirements for ethical research are met.

B-She should have reviewed the study protocol reviewed by ethics committee

C-The doctor should have asked for advice from colleagues familiar with research

D-She should always keep the patient's best interest in mind. If a patient is already benefitting from a treatment, assigning a patient to a placebo arm is unethical.

E-All the above

Confidentiality

As with patients in clinical care, research subjects have a right to privacy about health information.

Physician-patient relationship is different from the researcher's role in the researcher-research subject relationship, even if the physician and the researcher are the same person. The physician role must take precedence. The physician must be prepared to recommend that the patient not take part in a research project if the patient is doing well with current treatment and the project requires that patients be randomized to different treatments or to a placebo. Only if the physician, on solid scientific grounds, is truly uncertain whether the patient's current treatment is as suitable as a proposed new treatment, or even a placebo, should the physician ask the patient to take part in the research project.

Honest Reporting of Results

There have been many recent cases of dishonest practices in the publication of research results. Such practices may cause great harm to patients, who may be given incorrect treatments based on inaccurate or false research reports

Whistleblowing

Prevention of unethical research, or to expose it after the fact is an obligation. Whistleblowing is not always appreciated or even acted on, and whistle-blowers are sometimes punished or shunned for trying to expose wrongful acts. Government regulators are noticing the need to detect and punish unethical research and appreciate the role of whistle-blowers in reaching their targets.

Q-14 An 84-year-old Alzheimer's patient has been asked to participate in a clinical trial for a new drug designed to help improve memory. You were present when the clinical investigator obtained a signed informed consent from the patient a few days ago. Today when you see the patient and ask her about the study, she looks at you with a blank stare and has no idea what you are referring to.

What should be your next step?

A-The signed informed consent for the clinical drug testing is doubtful and should not proceed.

B-Contact the primary investigator to discuss the patient's participation in the trial.

C-A surrogate can give consent for her participation if the clinical trial is truly deemed to be in her best interests.

D-All the above are correct.

Q15 Preliminary analysis of results of a large clinical trial show that there were twice as many participants in the experimental group with gastrointestinal manifestations compared to the control group. Three of the cases required hospital admissions. However, the preliminary analysis reveals that there may be a moderate benefit with the new drug.

What should be done?

A. The adverse events are not serious enough to report.

B. The adverse events should be reported to the Data Safety Monitoring Board, and the serious adverse events must be reported to the IRB.

C. The large clinical trial should be stopped immediately.

D. Report in detail all the adverse events after completion of trial.

CHAPTER 12

Reportable Illnesses

The purpose in reporting illnesses is epidemiological in an attempt to interrupt the spread of certain communicable diseases. Reportable illnesses include AIDS, syphilis, tuberculosis, gonorrhea, and all childhood diseases such as measles, mumps, rubella, and pertussis.

Because of the social stigma associated with HIV, there is an additional layer of confidentiality and consent required. When a patient signs a release to distribute or transmit medical information, there is an additional consent required for HIV or AIDS-related information.

Physicians are legally protected in providing partner notification. The Department of Health takes charge of contact-tracing events and notifies those who have been in close contact with the source. The name of the source patient is always protected.

The Health Department can incarcerate patients with tuberculosis to prevent the spread of this disease, but such incarceration is not part of the judicial system and takes place at a hospital as a last resource to protect the public.

If a patient avoids disclosure to his or her partner, the physician must follow his/her duty to report to protect the innocent third party.

Gunshot Wounds

Reporting of gunshot wounds is mandatory, in pursuit of a criminal investigation, and despite a victim's objection. Safety of society takes precedence over patient privacy.

Q16 You have a pregnant HIV-positive patient in your office and ask her if she has informed her partner of her HIV status. In the past she had repeatedly resisted your attempts to inform the partner. Now she's pregnant with his child, sitting in the waiting room, and you have met him in the past?

What should you do?

A-respect for confidentiality

B-the refer patient to another physician

C- inform the partner immediately

D-respect the patient's confidentiality.

Q17A 26-year-old female is admitted to the hospital with irritability, severe headache, stiff neck and photophobia and mental status remains intact. Tests reveal Toxoplasmosis encephalitis cryptococcal an infection associated with HIV infection. Patient adamantly refuses to be tested for HIV.

How should you proceed in this case?

A-HIV testing despite the patient's refusal is a matter of public safety.

B-Avoid testing for HIV, as for any other medical procedure, testing should be done only with the informed consent of the patient.

C-Test the patient for HIV anonymously, without any identifying remarks.

D-Report the patient's toxoplasmosis to the Public Health Department

Q18 A 32-year-old man with AIDS is an active intravenous drug user. He keeps all his clinic appointments. He admits that he is unable to take his medications regularly when using drugs. He is asking your opinion on antiretroviral therapy with protease inhibitors. You recall that HIV viral resistance to protease inhibitors occurs when patients do not take their medications as directed.

Should you consider prescribing protease inhibitors to this patient?

A-Yes because the patient wants the protease inhibitors.

B-No because resistance is a real concern in a patient who cannot take his medicines timely.

C- No because the patient is continuing to use heroin and cocaine.

D- Yes, because the doctor is under a duty not to abandon the patient and to continue an ongoing therapeutic relationship. Patient must be provided with continued guidance and information about his HIV disease and issues of addiction.

CHAPTER 13

Physician as the Patient

1. A physician treating a patient who is also a physician must report if the physician-patient suffers from any medical condition where it is reasonably clear that patients of the physician-patient or others involved in his/her medical practice, could be harmed physically or psychologically as a result of the medical condition.

2. The treating physician must make reasonable efforts to determine the scope of the physician-patient's practice and seek information with consent from the physician-patient about the impact of the medical condition on the practice.

3. The physician-patient must be advised of their duty to self-report and must be supported in their reporting to the Medical Board.

4. The treating physician must advise the physician-patient of their intent to report.

CHAPTER 14

End of Life

Withholding-Withdrawal of Treatment

All adults with the capacity to understand their own medical conditions have the right to decide what treatments they wish to receive. There is no ethical or legal distinction between withholding and withdrawal of medical treatment.

There may be an emotional distinction between withholding respiratory assistance and stopping it after it has started, but there is no ethical distinction between the two.

When a treating physician suspects anxiety or depression, or any other mental health issue that may interfere with a patient's decision-making process, a psychiatric consult is prudent.

Withdrawing Treatment from Patients Without Decisional Capacity

It is important to note an important distinction between competence and decisional capacity.

Decisional capacity is a clinical determination that a patient's physician is medically qualified and legally authorized to make. Moreover, while many physicians seek a psychiatric consult (when readily available) prior to making such determinations, one is not required by law. Clinical literature also suggests, however, that the assessment of decisional capacity is not a skill that many physicians possess.

Diagnosis of depression does not preclude decisional capacity. When making such determinations, physicians should also be aware of a fundamental principle of American jurisprudence that every adult is presumed to possess decisional capacity, and the burden of persuasion falls upon anyone who asserts the contrary.

Q19 An 82-year-old white female is admitted with shortness of breath, hyperkalemia and metabolic acidosis. She has end-stage renal disease and based on the volume overload and emergency hemodialysis is indicated. Risks, benefits, and likelihood of death are discussed with the patient and she verbalizes understanding. She refuses dialysis and states, "I have had a good life and I am at peace with my lord." Her medical chart contains an advanced directive and appoints her son as the surrogate decision-maker. What should be your next step?

A-withhold hemodialysis

B- order hemodialysis

C- discuss hemodialysis with patient's son

D-assess the patient's decision-making capacity

Q20A 28-year-old male sustains a large subdural hematoma post motor vehicle accident. His oxygen saturation is dropping, and intubation is imminent. The patient's mother insists on all measures to be taken to save his life. However, the male partner is the healthcare agent. He reports that the patient had repeatedly stated that he would never want to be on a ventilator for any reason. What is the best next step?

    A- Obtain a full neurological evaluation
    B- Consult the ethics committee
    C- Honor the mother's wishes and intubate
    D- Honor the agent of proxy and do not intubate

Advance Directive

A method by which a patient communicates his wishes for his/her healthcare in advance of becoming unable to make decisions for him/herself. The advance directive is part of the concept of autonomy. Thus, last-minute decision-making processes, emotionally driven by family members, can be avoided.

Living Will, Health-Care Proxy

A living will is a written form of advance directive that outlines the care that a patient would want for him/herself if he/she were to lose the ability to communicate, or the capacity to understand his/her medical problems.

The living will is be usable when specific tests and treatments are outlined. A living will would overrule the wishes of the family, because the living will communicates the patient's own wishes. Unfortunately, living wills often lack specificity, and furthermore, most patients do not have an advance directive order. A united family often makes the decisions for the patient.

In absence of clear advance directive, and a family disagreement on what the patient wanted for himself or herself, the recourse is to refer to the ethics committee and the courts.

"Do Not Resuscitate" (DNR) Orders

A "Do Not Resuscitate" (DNR) order means, if the patient dies, not to perform CPR, cardioversion, or antiarrhythmics. "DNR" is not a declaration of pending death.

A patient should receive all necessary medical procedures, and DNR should be viewed purely as the endpoint of therapies. A DNR patient should receive all medical attention, all but CPR, etc.

Q21 A 68-year-old female presents to the emergency department with shortness of breath. Past medical history is significant for diabetes, coronary artery disease, and hypertension. She has a DNR/DNI status. Lab results reveal severe hyperkalemia and the patient is in renal failure.

What should be the next step?

A-Admit to the general medical floor with medications.

B-Dialyze the patient and admit to ICU, avoid intubation.

C-Inform the patient that the DNR/DNI does not allow him to be admitted to hospital.

D-Inform the patient that she needs to revoke her DNR/DNI status for treatment.

Q22 A 70-year-old man is admitted for acute appendicitis. This patient has a DNR status since his previous admission. He needs an urgent appendectomy. He still wishes to maintain the DNR. How should you explain the scenario to the patient?

A -Reverse the DNR order to attempt the surgery.

B -DNR is acceptable if there is no intubation.

C -DNR does not preclude surgery, proceed with anticipated surgery.

E -No surgery can be performed patient due to the patient's DNR status.

Q23 A 72-year-old patient advises his family that he would never want to be a vegetable attached to a breathing machine. What is the most likely perception of the treating physician?

A -The patient does not want any heroics measures.

B- Disconnect the respirator if the patient is ever in terminal state.

C- Allow the patient to die in a comatose state.

D-The physician should request more clarification for advanced care planning.

Q24- An elderly man with congestive heart failure presents to the emergency room alert and oriented complaining of shortness of breath. Chest X-Ray reveals that he has pneumonia. He starts desaturating in the emergency room and he has an impending respiratory failure, though still awake and alert. A copy of living will is in his chart clearly states that he wants no "invasive" medical procedures that may only prolong his death. Should mechanical ventilation be instituted?

A-A living will, or other advance directive obviates the responsibility to involve a competent patient in medical decision making.

B-An awake and alert patient overrides all advance directives, his living will is therefore irrelevant to medical decision making.

C-Risks and benefits of mechanical ventilation need not be presented to the patient because of the presence of a valid living will.

D-If the patient refuses mechanical ventilation therapy, his wishes should not be honored because he is in the emergency room.

Nutrition

The artificial administration of fluids and nutrition is a medical procedure and treatment that can be accepted or refused by a competent adult. "Artificial administration" basically refers to any form of nutrition other than eating through the mouth. "Artificial" specifically means feedings or fluids administered by nasogastric, gastric, or jejunostomy tube placement. "Artificial nutrition" and intravenously administered nutrition such as total parenteral nutrition is also referred to as hyperalimentation.

Patients who cannot speak are a challenge in medical decision making. Nutrition is the single most difficult issue in terms of treatment cessation. Physicians can never withhold simple nutrition like food to eat and water to drink. Hence, clear evidence of a patient's wishes regarding artificial nutrition is clearly important. Again, a lack of clarity in a patient's wishes mandates a referral to the Ethics Committee.

Futile Care

Treatments, investigations, and tests must ultimately benefit the patient, and should not be administered to satisfy the curiosity of family members. <u>Certainty</u> in withholding or withdrawing therapy based on futility is paramount.

Q25 An elderly man residing in a nursing home is admitted to the medical floor with pneumonia. He is awake but grossly demented. He can only utter sound yet interacts and acknowledges family members. The admitting resident states that treating his pneumonia with antibiotics would be "futile" and suggests informing the family.

What is the proper approach?

A-Treating the patient's pneumonia with antibiotics stands a reasonable chance of success.

B-Patient is severely demented, treating his pneumonia with antibiotics would be "futile".

C-The treatment of pneumonia in this severely demented patient is futile because antibiotics may be ineffective.

D-None of the above.

Physician Assisted Suicide

In physician-assisted suicide, the physician provides the patient with the means of ending his/her own life. The physician does not actually administer the substance that ends the patient's life. Despite much controversy around the topic, physician-assisted suicide is considered unethical.

Euthanasia

Euthanasia means that the healthcare worker is prescribing and administering the method of death. In the United States, euthanasia is illegal.

Terminal Sedation

Intentional high-dose opiates in order to end a patient's life is wrong, but it is acceptable to give pain medications even if they might decrease a patient's respiratory drive, in order to ultimately decrease pain and suffering. A physician cannot leave a patient to simply suffer, as the ethical duty is to relieve pain. The key, of course, is the intention behind the chosen course of action.

Organ Donation

Organ donation is a voluntary act. No one, and no court of law, has jurisdiction to mandate organ donation.

The organ donor network should obtain consent for an organ donation, not the medical team, as the priority of the medical team is not to obtain organs.

Organ donor cards provide the healthcare team with an indication of a patient's wishes for donation. Family members' objections can overrule the organ donor card.

Q26 A 44-year-old male responds to an ad, where he is offered a large sum for his kidney. This will help him with his desperate financial dilemma. He is requesting a full medical evaluation to be approved for the procedure.

What should be your response?

A-It is unacceptable to receive any money for solid organs donation.

B-It is acceptable if the recipient is in true need for the organ.

C-It is okay if the donor's remaining kidney is healthy.

D-Profiting from the donation is unacceptable.

Q27 A man arrives at the hospital post a crushing MVA; he meets all criteria as brain-dead. He has an organ donor card indicating his wishes to donate. The organ donor team contacts the family. The family refuses to sign a consent for donation.

What should be immediate considerations?

A-Seek a court order to overrule family.

B-Honor family's wishes against donation.

C-Remove the organs, regardless of family's wishes.

D-Wait for complete cardiac arrest, then remove the organs.

CHAPTER 15

Doctor and Society

Culture Awareness

A physician's humility should extend to recognize diversity, cultural values, orientation and their significance in a patient's decision-making process. The physician should also identify some basic familiarity with today's diverse cultures.

A physician should not assume that a patient exercises all beliefs of an ethnic or racial community. Asking appropriate questions will help to identify the patient's beliefs and values.

Child Abuse

All physicians have a duty to report child abuse with no discretion. There is no discretion on whether to report abuse. Even suspected child abuse must be reported, and reporting to child protective services should be prompt, to prevent further abuse. If a report is being sincerely and honestly made, there is no associated liability.

Elder Abuse

The circumstances with elder abuse are less clear than child abuse, because an elderly person is often an adult who may object to the report of abuse, as they fear repercussions at home, or even loss of the home. Nevertheless, you must report the abuse to adult protective services.

Q28 An 86-year-old female presents to the office for follow-up care. Patient has several abrasions and ecchymoses and has been losing weight. She is widowed and lives with her granddaughter and her husband. Through further questioning, she does admit that her granddaughters' husband occasionally physically abuses her when he is drunk. What should be done?

A-meet with you patient and granddaughters' husband.

B - engage home healthcare agency to evaluate home situation.

C- have the patient removed from the house placed in an adult home environment.

D- Reported grandson in law to adult protective services.

E - Report the abuse only with patients' consent.

Duty to Warn

A physician must have reasonable grounds to warn possible victim if a patient may be in danger of harming others. Duty to warn is one of the few exceptions to the patient's right to confidentiality. In cases of homicidal or suicidal ideation, the practitioner has a moral and legal obligation to inform potential victims and the proper authorities.

Q29 You are the primary care to a patient with a history of schizophrenia. During a follow up visit, he informs you of his frustrations with his boss. He asks if everything during the office visit is confidential, and you state that it is, in response. He then states "Sometimes, I really think that I will kill my boss if I get a chance."

What should be your next step?

A-Inform the patient's boss of the threat

B-inform law enforcement of the threat to the patient's boss

C-continue to discourage patient of his plan and maintain confidentiality

D-inform both the patient's boss and law enforcement of the threat

E-Commit patient to the psychiatric ward.

CHAPTER 16

Reproductive Issues

Abortion

An adult woman has an unrestricted right to abortion through the end of the first trimester. In the second trimester, the decision is still between a woman and her attending physician, but the ease of access is not so clear. States may place regulations on access to a second-trimester abortion. However, second-trimester abortions are still performed at the patient's discretion. Third-trimester abortions are not available since the fetus is viable, and are clearly restricted. The father's consent for an abortion is not required. The fetus is considered as a part of the woman's body and does not have the individual rights of 'personhood' until after birth.

It is unethical for a patient to seek an abortion for gender selection. Fundamentally, if there is a procedure that a patient wants which appears unethical, you should refer the patient to another physician. The physician must voluntarily agree to the physician-patient relationship.

Contraception

Contraception has no limitation and is entirely at the discretion of the patient. This is equally true for minors. Contraception is one of the issues for which a minor is considered partially emancipated. Parental consent is not necessary to obtain contraception.

Q30 A young couple present to your office to discuss contraception. The wife wishes to have tubal ligation. Her husband is shocked and upset stating that they have no children and storms out of the room. The wife is adamant about sterilization and wishes to move forward with the procedure.

What should be next?

    A- Proceed with a psychological evaluation.
    B- Proceed with tubal ligation
    C- Refer only with husband's consent
    D- Schedule a follow up appointment to reevaluate the decision

Sterilization

Men and women have free access to sterilization. Consent is only necessary from the patient. Each patient has autonomy over his or her own body.

CHAPTER 17

Impaired Drivers

All states require patients to report seizure disorders or visual acuity changes. Nationally, there is no consensus amongst states in regard to reporting practices. The Department of Motor Vehicles (DMV) is the only authority which can suspend or revoke driving privileges. Drivers should take it upon themselves to report any relevant impairments to the DMV, and physicians should encourage all impaired drivers to limit their driving. Physicians cannot suspend driving privileges.

Q32 An 88-year-old male patient presents to the office in a follow-up minor MVA where he hit the left side of his head. He renewed his driver's license two years ago and his only restriction is wearing glasses. You have concerns about patient safety if he continues to drive. What should be done?

A –neurological examination and evaluation

B – imaging of the brain

C- revoke patient's license to drive

D- discussed the matter with the family to prevent him from driving

E-discussed the matter with the patient and encourage him to stop driving since this may put him and others in danger, remind him that there are always other means of transportation.

CHAPTER 18

Impaired Physician

Doctors also have an obligation to report impaired physicians to authorities for treatment.

A Physician must report another Physician when it is believed that the conduct of his/her colleague places patients at risk or is considered unprofessional or unethical.

Reportable categories include suffering from a physical, cognitive, mental, or emotional condition that is negatively impacting the work of the Physician and the work environment, and sexually inappropriate advances, a sexual relationship with a patient, or any sexual boundary violations. An impaired physician should be treated with equal dignity and respect offered to any patient.

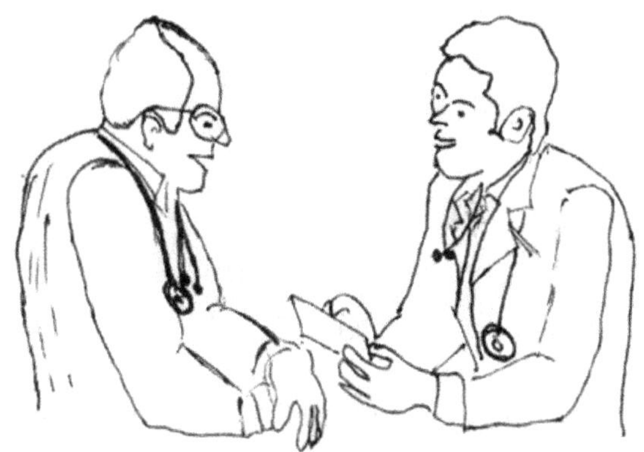

Ultimately, if a complaint is made from a patient to another Physician about sexual boundary violation, a physician must guide the patient on how to file a complaint, even if they wish to remain anonymous

Q32 Your 68-year-old colleague is noted to be forgetful with staff names, patient's names and frequently misses hospital meetings. You're concerned about your colleague's cognitive status. What would be the next best step?

A-offer to evaluate the colleague in confidence

B-approach the colleague and help him plan for confidential evaluation

C-continue to monitor the colleague a while longer

D-report the colleague to the medical board anonymous

Q33 A physician is noted to yell at a floor nurse and leaving the floor. Recently, he has been observed engaging in uncharacteristic behavior. During a recent pharma educational dinner, he was drinking heavily and was unruly at times. His appearance also has been disheveled.

Which is the best course of action for a colleague?

A- Interview the physician's staff about his recent behavior

B- Inquiry from other physicians about similar conduct

C- Question the nurse about the physician's outburst

D- Notify the chief of medicine

CHAPTER 18

Spousal Abuse

Abuse against a patient can only be reported with the consent of the patient. Many victims feel they are not able to leave their relationships or to report the abuse as they fear retaliation. Counselling should be offered to the patient.

Q34 A 52-year-old female presents to the office for follow up. She has multiple contusions and a black eye. She admits that her husband beats her. You state that you will have to report this to authorities. She adamantly states that she does not want her injuries reported.

What is the next step?

A-You will report the injury only with consent.

B-You agree not to report, unless there is another episode.

C-You must report as reporting is mandatory.

D-You have to ascertain that physical abuse came from the husband.

CHAPTER 19

Elder Abuse

Mistreatment of the elderly has become a matter of public concern over the past few decades. Mistreatment of older persons may occur both within home and community settings, and institutional environments. The definition of elder abuse and neglect is a matter of state law, and each state has its own statutory schema.

The National Research Council has described elder mistreatment as:

(a) intentional actions that cause harm or create a serious risk of harm (whether harm is intended) to a vulnerable elder by a caregiver or other person who stands in a trusted relationship to the elder or

(b) failure of a caregiver to satisfy the elder's basic needs or to protect the elder from harm.

Elder mistreatment is physical (e.g., assault, forced sexual contact, overmedication, inappropriate physical restraints); psychological, or emotional. This includes denial of basic human needs by the caregiver (e.g., withholding indicated medical care or food), deprivation of civil rights (e.g., freedom of movement and communication), and financial exploitation.

In addition, a significant proportion of reported cases of elder mistreatment fall into the category of self-neglect where older persons are living alone. Self-neglect may be suspected in the presence of dehydration, malnourishment, decubitus ulcers, poor personal hygiene, or lack of compliance with basic medical recommendations.

In recognition of the potential for elder abuse and neglect, states have created a wide variety of programs under the general heading of Adult Protective Services (APS). This is a system of preventive and supportive services for older persons living in the community to enable them to remain as independent as possible, while avoiding abuse and exploitation by others.

CHAPTER 20

Gifts from the Industry

AMA medical ethics II stipulates gifts to Physicians from any industry creates conditions that carry the risk of subtly biasing—or being perceived to bias—professional judgment in the care of patients.

To preserve the trust that is fundamental to the patient-physician relationship and public confidence in the profession, physicians should:

(a) Decline cash gifts in any amount from an entity that has a direct interest in physicians' treatment recommendations.

(b) Decline any gifts for which reciprocity is expected or implied.

(c) Accept an in-kind gift for the physician's practice only when the gift will directly benefit patients, including patient education, and is of minimal value

(d) Academic institutions and residency and fellowship programs may accept special funding on behalf of trainees to support medical students', residents', and fellows' participation in professional meetings, including educational meetings, provided:

1. The program identifies recipients based on independent institutional criteria
2. Funds are distributed to recipients without specific attribution to sponsors.

Gifts from Patients

Small gifts from patients of modest value are acceptable on the part of the physician, if there is no expectation of a different form of therapy, or a higher level of care.

Cakes and cookies for Christmas, a birthday card or balloon on a birthday, or other tokens of gratitude are acceptable.

CHAPTER 21

Prescribing Opiates, or Not

A physician must be able to justify prescribing decisions with documentary evidence of a patient's initial assessment and reassessments as required, including when accepting the transfer of care of a patient from another healthcare provider.

CDC Guidelines (March 2016)

- Nonpharmacologic therapy should be attempted as the primary treatment

- Opioids should be continued only if improvement in pain and function outweighs risk.

- Clinicians should discuss known risks and realistic benefits of opioid therapy and managing therapy with patients

- Start with immediate-release opioids, and use the lowest effective dosage

- Limit quantities for short term therapy and assess efficacy of opioids regularly. If no benefit is perceived, taper or stop.

- Evaluate for risk factors.

- Access prescription drug monitoring programs for refills

- Use urine drug testing.

- Avoid concurrent use of opiates and benzodiazepines

- Use buprenorphine or methadone in combination with behavioral therapies for patients with opioid-use disorder.

At the time of initial assessment, a physician must discuss and determine with the patient the best medication choice considering the:

(a)   efficacy of other pharmacological and non-pharmacological treatment options.

(b)   common and potentially serious side effects of the medication; and

(c)   probability the medication will improve the patient's health and function.

The physician must review the patient's medication history from PMP, before initiating and renewing a prescription, at minimum every month when the prescription is for the long-term treatment of a patient. In the event of inaccessible PMP or lack of a patient's medication history, physicians should prescribe the minimum amount of medication required until more information can be obtained.

A physician who prescribes long-term opioid treatment for a patient with chronic pain, or as exclusive treatment for active cancer, palliative or end-of-life care, must also have a pain management contract signed by the patient and the physician, and this contract must be fully explained to the patient, with an executed copy provided. A violation of the pain management contract is grounds for dismissal from a pain management agreement, i.e. any further opiate prescription. Furthermore, a spot urine toxicology screen, serves as a tool for patient compliance.

It is important to:

(a) Establish and measure goals for function and pain for the patient,

(b) Evaluate and document risk factors for opioid-related harms,

(c) Prescribe the lowest effective dose and, doses that exceed the opioid prescribing guidelines should be carefully justified and clearly documented in patient's chart,

(d) Reassess the patient within four weeks of initiating opiates and every four weeks thereafter,

(e) Document the status of the patient's function and pain at each reassessment; and

(f) Renew opiates only if there is a measurable clinical improvement in function and pain that justifies the risks of continued opioid treatment

Patient Drug Abuse warning signs:

1.Declines a physical exam and diagnostic tests, and won't allow the physician to obtain past records

2. Travels an exceedingly long distance or out of state for the visit without explanation

3. Seeks medications from emergency rooms, urgent care facilities or walk-in clinics

4. Has prescriptions from multiple providers without the physician's knowledge

(Access available via Prescription Drug Monitoring Programs)

5. Resists changes in the treatment plan despite evidence of adverse effects.

6. Repeated claims of lost prescription or medication.

7. Declines non-pharmacologic therapies

8. Attempts to change, forge, or rewrite prescriptions.

9. Diverts or sells medication or borrows drugs from others

10. Requests prescriptions written in the names of other people

CHAPTER 22

<u>Telemedicine and Telecommunicating with Patient</u>

Telemedicine is defined as medical diagnosis and patient care through electronic media where the patient and the provider are in different locations. The technology's potential to enhance value-based care has contributed to the widespread adoption of telemedicine. A licensed physician in one state cannot treat a patient across state lines, unless said physician also holds a license for the state where the patient resides. Otherwise, practicing in a state without a medical license has serious legal implications.

Important considerations for telemedicine include:

-Do not start practicing telemedicine without a written informed consent specifically for platform used,

- Know the location of the patient before treatment - are you licensed in the state where the patient is located?

- Determine what your role is with this patient. Diagnosing? Therapy? Treatment? Evaluation? Consulting?

-Are you licensed in the state the patient is located?

-The standard of care does not change with telemedicine, and is equivalent to an in-person clinical visit

-A business associates' agreement is necessary if information is stored in any way for any amount of time by your technology vendor.

-You must require audit trails from your business associate, and they must be contractually required to notify you of any privacy breaches

-check with state law and licensing board requirements for compatibility and encryption requirements for your system

-Ensure compatibility with payer requirements, including Medicaid and Medicare, and other approved vendors.

-Be aware of state laws on telemedicine where the patient is living, and if treating a patient in another state you must know clinical legal standards that apply to the patient's location.

-You must have a reliable and HIPAA compliance system in place

Q35 A 27-year-old female is using the telemedicine services for the first time. She is connected to the telemedicine doctor from her cubicle at the office. Her medical records are not available. The patient has had a few days of a productive cough, headache and inability to have a good night sleep due her spastic cough and associated fatigue. Dr. Eager suggests an infection of her lungs.The patient reports feeling uncomfortable, has many deadlines to meet for work and is not able to leave work. "I had a similar infection last year, and I would appreciate calling in an antibiotic."

The physician requests an in person visit, for a full exam and chest x-ray.The patient hangs up frustrated. The physician is frustrated with the interaction and fears that his compensation could be negatively affected by exercising proper clinical judgement.

What would have improved the outcome?

A-Restructure the reimbursement not to affect standard of care.

B-Educate the patient further regarding standard of care to improve her health

C-Provide the patient with a sick note, to manage her work deadlines till she is seen in person.

D- Speak to patient's primary care giver to obtain history.

E-All the above

Email:

You must have a written informed consent specifically for email usage with a patient, and your first email (unless in response to the patient) should be without a message, with the word "test" as the subject line. Educate patients about the need for security and password protection for their devices, and if uncomfortable with e-communications with a client, seek alternative means of communication. Patients must be made understand the pitfalls of email.

It is important to ensure a HIPAA compliant encrypted email system is in place, and avoid using a patient's name, nicknames, protected information, or record identifiers within emails, including, but not limited to:

- Address, ZIP Code, birth date, admission dates and age.
- Phone or fax number, photographic image, Social Security number.
- Information about mental illness, developmental disabilities, communicable diseases, substance abuse, sexual assault, child abuse, and medical illnesses.

CHAPTER 23

Social Media

Social media is a serious challenge for physicians. As both doctors and patients exchange thoughts and stories on Facebook, Instagram, and other social media platforms, this opens a portal to risky consequences, including:

- Excess: People tend to lose normal inhibitions online and end up saying things they would never say in person. Once said, it is no longer yours to control, and can be legally used against you.

- Who is on the other side: When sending emails and texts, one has no idea who can access them.

- State lines: Recommendations you offer online can be passed on to other states. You can be charged with practicing without a license, if you are not licensed in those states.

- Staff: A physician is responsible for his/her staff's actions. If a staff member posts a photo or comment that violates the law, the physician will be the one who will be disciplined.

- Becoming too friendly with patients: Physicians who share too much personal information with patients online are basically allowing patients to get personally closer to them, which is outside of professional conduct.

Q35 A multispecialty physician group hired a new graduate, who is well liked by patients and staff alike, and her clinical care is excellent. A senior physician in the group discovers the new physician's social media page contains negative remarks about obese patients and non-compliant patients without naming any names. She also has many photos at parties, drinking alcohol, and behaving unprofessionally. What is the most appropriate course of action?

A-Advise the most senior physician in the group about the post

B-Comment on social media about colleague's unprofessional conduct

C-Meet the colleague, discuss the inappropriate content and urge her to remove it.

D-No action is required.

CHAPTER 24

Managed Care

The term "managed care is" used in the United States to describe activities intended to reduce the cost of providing ***for-profit*** healthcare and provide health insurance while improving the quality of that care. Managed care plans are a type of health insurance, which include contracts with healthcare providers, medical facilities, and physicians to provide care for their members at reduced costs. These providers make up the plan's network, and how much of the care provided is paid for by the plan, depends on the network's rules.

Plans that restrict choices usually cost less, while more flexible plans cost more. There are three types of managed care plans:

- Health Maintenance Organizations (HMO) generally pay for care within a set network of physicians. The patient chooses a primary care doctor who coordinates most of his/her care.
- Preferred Provider Organizations (PPO) usually pay more of the cost of care if the care is within the network. PPOs still pay part of the cost if the care is outside of the network.
- Point of Service (POS) plans allow the patient to choose between an HMO or a PPO model each time care is needed.

CHAPTER 25

Medicine and the Law

Risk Management

Risk management is used to minimize the incidence of problematic behavior that might result in injury to patients and employees, and to decrease liability for the physician or the facility. The key element in risk management is identifying problem behaviors and practices in an organization such as a hospital or medical office. A plan should be formulated to eliminate these behaviors. Risk management factors across categories include wet floors, faulty equipment, clerical errors, poor record keeping, mishandling drugs and needles, poor patient follow up, and abandonment of patients.

Everyone in a healthcare facility is responsible for risk management.

Incident Report

An incident report is used to document problem areas within a medical facility.

Whenever there is an occurrence such as a fall, error in medication dispensing, potential contamination from a used needle, flood, fire, hazardous material leak, a patient or employee complaint must be documented within an incident reportby a physician, employee, or a manager.

The purpose of the report is to document exactly what happened, when it happened, and what was done to resolve the incident. This practice aims to prevent recurrences of such incidents.

Q36 You are a second-year resident on the general medical floor towards the end of your shift. After reviewing the chart for one of your patients, Tom, an insulin-dependent diabetic with heart failure, you forget to document administering his dose of insulin. During the night the patient receives another dose of insulin by the night shift staff. The following day while rounding on your patient he complains of having a very difficult night with profuse sweating headaches and feeling dizzy. You realize your error after reviewing the chart. You consult your attending physician who advises you to fill out an incident form. What should you tell Tom?......

A-claim that the nursing staff made an error

B-advise the patient of your mistake

C- apologize to the patient for the hardship and admit to making a mistake and assure him that you will take measures that this type of error never happens again.

D- request to meet with the ethics committee of the hospital

Q37 An 88-year-old man was admitted to the ICU one week ago with multiorgan failure and severe pneumonia. Weaning the patient off the ventilator has been futile as he continues to be unresponsive. His past medical history is significant for chronic kidney disease, hypertension, congestive heart failure, dementia, and diabetes type II. The medical team approaches the family and informs them that the patient will not have a meaningful recovery. The patient has no advance directives and his children insist on ICU level care.

Which is the most appropriate management?

A-Discontinue ICU care in 24 hours if no improvement.

B-Transfer patient to hospice

C-Refer the case to hospital ethics committee

D- Ask the patient's children to reconsider the facts.

CHAPTER 26

Medical Malpractice and Professional Liability

Merriam Webster dictionary defines malpractice as:

1: a dereliction of professional duty or a failure to exercise an ordinary degree of professional skill or learning by one (such as a physician) rendering professional services which results in injury, loss, or damage

2: an injurious, negligent, or improper practice: malfeasance

Treatments and procedures are conducted with the best intentions, and unfortunately, despite best efforts, the outcomes do not always turn out as expected. Sadly, we live in a litigious society, and in the case of medical incidents, patients and families need to hold someone responsible. Healthcare professionals are responsible not only for their actions, but those of their staff as well. Everyone associated with negligence is liable for damages.

Most cases reflect legal action against physicians, however all individuals in the medical profession can be sued.

There are "four Ds" to prove in malpractice litigation: **D**ereliction of **D**uty **D**irectly causing **D**amages.

Physicians encounter difficult situations every day in clinical practice and rely on the law for speedy guidance. Law demands obedience and punishes disobedience. Understanding legal rules and regulations, and adherence to this framework, provides clinicians with certain immunities against civil and criminal liability. However, in healthcare, when moral issues arise, the law is rather silent, which allows for choices to be made in healthcare for a patient or clinician.

Laws are not flawless, and healthcare professionals have a moral responsibility to protect their patients from harm, while also protecting themselves from liabilites. Absolute self-protection should not be the overriding factor, as any therapeutic modality poses a legal risk.

The American Medical Association's "Principles of Medical Ethics" states, "A physician shall respect the law and recognize a responsibility to seek changes in those requirements which are contrary to the best interests of the patient."

Q38 A 22-year-old female is admitted to the hospital with Steven Johnson Syndrome. Two weeks prior to admission, the patient was seen in the outpatient clinic by a colleague, and she was prescribed trimethoprim-sulfamethoxazole for a UTI. The patient's medical record clearly indicates that she has a sulfa allergy. The patient is clearly upset and expresses concern as to why she was prescribed a sulfa drug. What should be the next appropriate response?

    A- Offer to transfer patient care to another facility

    B- Reassure patient that prescribing physician will be informed, and steps will be taken to avoid future errors

    C- The patient's pharmacy is at fault for not detecting the error

    D-Arrange for the patient to meet the prescribing physician

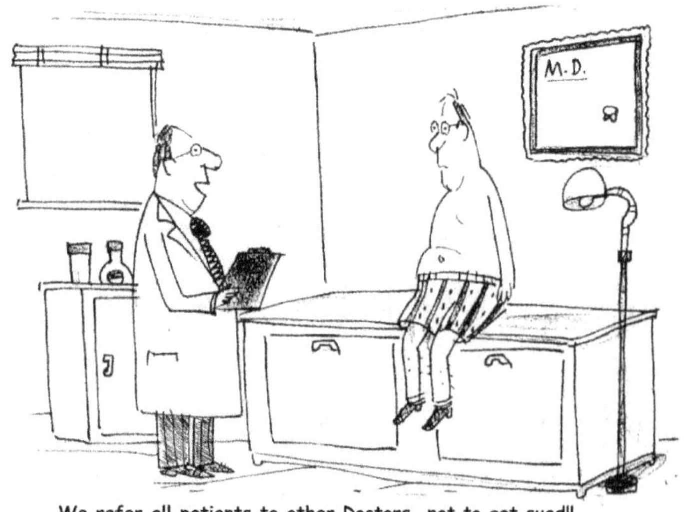

We refer all patients to other Doctors, not to get sued!!

CHAPTER 27

Risk Avoidance

It is important to note the following:

- Confidentiality does not "die" with the patient.

- Every clinician is required to maintain a record on every patient.

- You should always inquire of new patients as to whether they are involved in, or plan on becoming involved in, litigation that may include you.

  - Don't write anything in a patient's record that you would not want them to see.
  - Never write a letter on behalf of a patient that you could not defend in a court of law.
  - Never agree to refrain from maintaining a record on a patient.
  - Never change a record without making such change in a manner that will be transparent to anyone who reads it later.

Clinicians are <u>not</u> required either ethically or legally, to treat every patient that presents for treatment.

There are times when the clinician-patient relationship should be terminated for the benefit of the patient as well as the clinician.

The difference between a proper termination and a claim of abandonment is related to the process of termination. Abandonment is usually a precipitous act without notice to the patient or lacking a valid explanation. A proper termination involves a dialogue with the patient usually resulting in a transfer of the patient to a new provider.

In a psychotherapeutic relationship, gifts and compliments should be kept to a bare minimum; both in quality and quantity.

When a psychiatrist allows a patient's outstanding bill to accumulate to a level where the patient is angry over the amount, the fault no longer lies with the patient.

Prescriptions may only be written for legitimate medical purposes. This requires a clinician-patient relationship, and a medical history and exam. Medication prescribed by a physician should be warranted by, and consistent with, the diagnosis, and maintenance of a medical record is of utmost importance.

Physicians should never provide samples of medication to a patient without first placing the sample medications in a container with the physician's name and address, patient's name, name of the drug, dosage, strength per dosage unit, directions for use, and any cautionary statements.

CHAPTER 28

Boundary Violation

Boundaries create a therapeutic distance between physician and patient and clarify their respective roles and expectations. Boundaries define limits of the therapeutic relationship.

Most boundary determinations are seen daily in clinical practices. Physicians need to exercise judgement and apply ethical principles to manage the outcome of every such case.

Maintaining boundaries do not stop at the office or clinic setting. A patient may recognize you in a shopping mall and hug you or may send an expensive pen as an apology for his/her previous behavior. Or, the physician may be sitting on a bar stool at a local restaurant and his/her patient appears beside him/her and asks to buy him/her drink. What does one do in such a scenario?

Boundary violations of a sexual or financial nature will involve an ethics committee, attorneys, licensing boards, or ultimately, judge and jury. Physicians are responsible for making decisions in their patient's best interest at all times.

Clinicians must consider the vulnerabilities and risk factors and do what they can to increase accountability. This book is an attempt to help explain important prevention measures for such cases.

The adult who has never learned to say "no" becomes the doctor who is more interested in pleasing his/her patients, than using sound clinical judgment. The adolescent who has learned to manipulate others for his/her own end, can become the predatory physician who misuses his/her power over vulnerable patients.

Many physicians learn the wrong lessons on the job. Even the most well-adjusted professional, with a mature grasp of personal boundaries, does not enter the profession with a clear understanding of professional boundaries. The responsible physician must learn these unique boundaries sooner rather than later. It is difficult to learn the importance of establishing and respecting boundaries when those around you often disregard them, without any disciplinary actions.

Boundary violations do not just happen. They often begin slowly, and progress slowly enough to avoid detection—and then, it is too late. A physician may fantasize about a patient, and when no action has been taken, or no harm done, he/she remains within his/her sphere as this is not a violation. However, this behavior may drift to dangerous territories of violation.

A physician must avoid these mine fields, as a license to practice medicine is not an entitlement. License to practice medicine is only a privilege which physicians are trusted with and should always treasure and protect.

CHAPTER 29

National Practitioner Data Bank

Since 1990, the state medical and dental boards have been required to report certain disciplinary actions taken against the professionals they license to the National Practitioner Data Bank. Professional societies, too, must report adverse actions taken against their members, while insurers must report all malpractice payments. The U.S. Department of Health and Human Services makes this information available to state licensure boards and certain healthcare entities to facilitate the tracking of professionals who are disciplined in one state, then seek licensure in another. Healthcare facilities must query the Data Bank at least every two years regarding each member of their staff.

Many states now post this information on public websites as well, allowing patients to consider the legal history of practitioners when choosing a healthcare provider.

CHAPTER 30

State Medical Boards

The medical board's duty is to protect the public, not the physician. State medical boards today focus on licensed physicians who violate professional ethics, and their mandate has significantly evolved to focus on disciplining physicians.

The state defines the license to practice medicine as a privilege, not a right, and the state medical board that grants a license can also revoke it. If the board, for any reason, suspects, a lack of professionalism in serving patients in a safe manner, the medical license is at risk.

Disciplinary Action

Physicians who hold their positions in society are invited to respond to patient complaints in a very subtle manner. This invitation unfolds in a way which strips the physician of everything they have worked for all their lives, and their dignity and pride are often seemingly shattered.

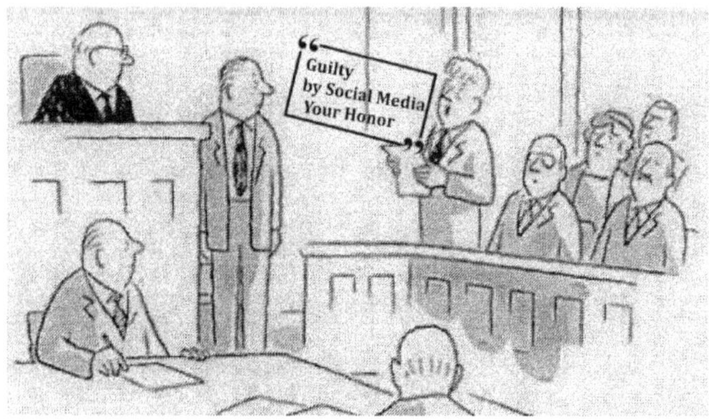

Unfortunately, the medical boards do not always use proper discretion with regards to media and release of information before a full investigation. Thus, the media has a field day, and it is open season on the physician and their families.

Boards are under increasing pressure to discipline violators. Ultimately, it is the board that makes the final decision, not the physician, and legal counsel serves as a witness to ensure a proper administrative procedure. Legal Counsel may present evidence on a physician's behalf, and will be heard, but again, the board makes the final decision, and is not to be compared with civil courts.

Complaints against the physician can come from any source: patients, employees, hospitals, and pharmacists, to name a few. The medical board will primarily side with the patient, regardless of patients' actions which may have led to the physician violation. The board may suspend a medical license until a hearing can be held, and if the violation appears severe, the board may choose to investigate using their investigative team, in the same manner and authority as a criminal investigation by the police. The board will work closely with state, federal, and local law enforcement when they deem necessary.

Once the board files a charge the physician and his/her attorney can request a conference. If a settlement is reached, the board will issue a consent order which precludes any appeals. Most physicians choose consent orders, as they are the quickest, least expensive path and allows them to get back on track. However, this settlement will be public record and may increase malpractice rates, and lead to being blacklisted with many insurance companies as payors.

In case a settlement is not agreed upon, a formal hearing will follow. An administrative judge presides over the hearing, where witnesses are questioned by both sides, and evidence is presented. The presiding judge does not hold the final decision but issues a recommendation which the board votes to accept or reject. Keep in mind, this is not a civil court, and there is no presumption of innocence. So, no matter how convinced one is that an accuser lacks proof for charges and that the evidence is in one's favor, it is the board that will ultimately decides. There are limited rights of appeal, and they often prove to be unsuccessful.

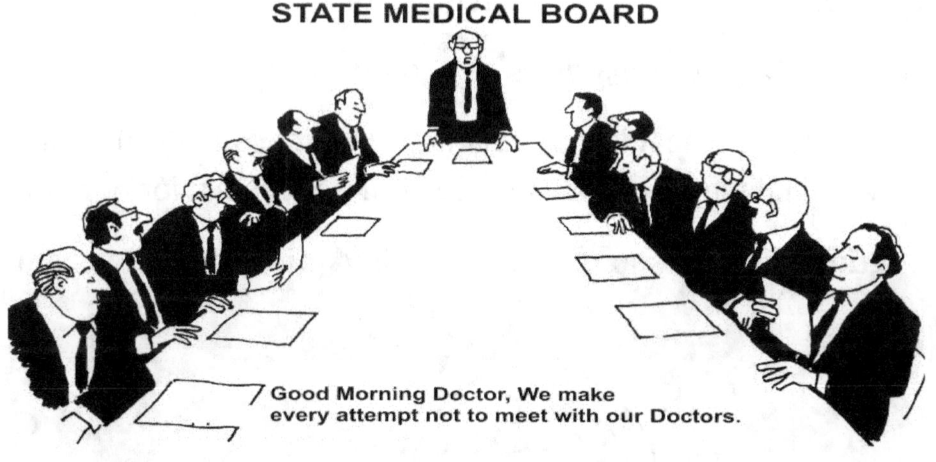

Most physicians disciplined by the boards are convinced they have been treated unfairly. Over the years, the disciplined physicians succumb to the 5 stages of grief: denial, anger, bargaining, depression, and finally acceptance, that the ultimate decision regarding their livelihood lies with the state medical boards.

Medical boards may suspend a license for a period, or completely revoke it. Whether the violation is minor, which may lead to fines, or a formal reprimand, a physician's license is not affected until a true suspension or revocation.

The medical board may require the physician to complete continuing medical education courses, or be evaluated for competency and medical aptitude, or undergo treatment at a state Physicians Health Program, before reentering medical practice. The return to practice may also be conditional, involving a mentor or a practice monitoring agency, or by having designated chaperones. Chaperones should be considered akin to medical malpractice insurance and having a chaperone at every visit provides the physician with a live witness. The medical board can revoke a license if the restrictions put forth are not followed.

Make no mistake: members of the medical board are regular people of different professions who may live next door. One of them may be an attorney, a doctor, nurse, engineer, social worker, or a businessperson, and they all have established opinions on ethics.

- The board's duty is to protect the public, never the physician

- The board always sides with patients, known as "vulnerable parties"

- Boundaries are open to board interpretation.

- There is no consensual sex between a doctor and a patient.

- Patient trust is a professional duty and a condition of licensure.

- A "dual relationship" with a patient jeopardizes objectivity.

- The physician is responsible for managing the relationship with patients, the staff, and anyone involved in any way in the medical practice, regardless of behavior or motivations.

- **Avoid disciplinary actions: once it starts, it does not end, and you will become a target.**

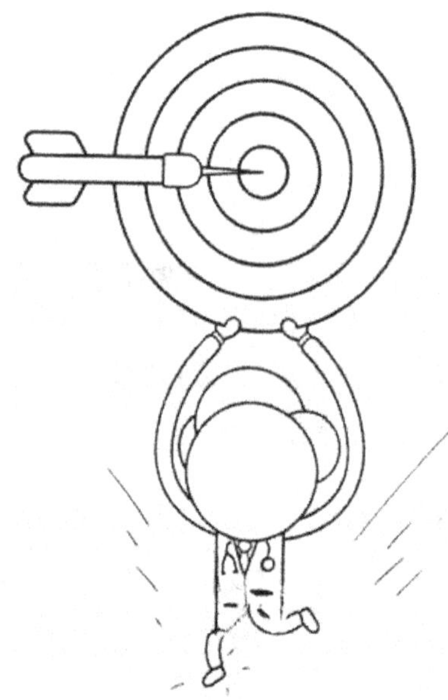

<u>**Answers to Questions**</u>

Q1-D In the absence of a formal advance directive, previously expressed wishes of a patient takes precedence.

Q2- D Mother has autonomy over what happens to her body, despite fetal rights in the third trimester.

Q3- A Asking a patient's treatments explained a comprehension and the consequences of the treatment should be ascertained. An appropriate criterion for a burdensome treatment is to not only ask what a patient wants, but why he or she chooses a treatment choice.

Q4- A This is an emergency, and treatment can be given in the patient's best interest. Consent is implied in an emergency.

Q5- A This patient is aware of the consequences of treatment refusal. As he is competent to make this decision, you must respect his wishes.

Q6- A Confidentiality involves respecting the privacy and wishes of a patient, and a physician should not release a patient's personal medical information without his or her consent. Exceptions to this policy may occur to protect individuals or the public or to disclose or report information as required by law.

Q7-C The content of medical record belongs to the patient and has every right to request a copy.

Q8-B, Physicians are ethically and legally obligated to disclose medical errors to patients.

Q9-D, You must establish a physician-patient relationship before engaging.

Q10-D This is a difficult situation. The most ethical way is to send a letter, certified, copy to chart and signature requested. What if the letter comes back to your office? Are you obligated to refill renewal requests from the pharmacy?

Q11-B Physicians are accountable for their behavior. Appropriate measure should be taken through formal channels if inappropriate behavior is not corrected.

Q12-B Patients genetic testing is confidential and can only be releases with patient authorization. The employer has no right to a patients' genetic information.

Q13-C Knowledge of the protocol submitted to the ethics review committee and any comments or conditions is mandatory. She should ensure that she act is in the best interests of her patients and enrolls those who will not be harmed by changing their current stable treatment to the experimental one or to placebo. She should never agree to a fixed number of patient enrollment, since this leads to pressure patients enrol. She should carefully monitor the patients in the study for adverse events and to adopt corrective action. She should communicate the results of the research to her patients as they become available.

Q14-D The competence of patient for a valid informed consent is doubtful. You should contact the primary investigator to discuss participation in the trial. Although the patient belongs to the population under study, and her participation may benefit herself and other Alzheimer's patients. However, a careful balancing of risks and benefits must be considered.

Q15-B All adverse events are reported to the Data Safety Monitoring Board, and serious adverse events must be reported to the IRB. Investigators should consider reevaluating the balance of risks versus benefits. These findings may draw each participant's willingness to continue in the trial, and according to 45 CFR 46.116(b)(5) the findings should be provided to all current and future participants as part of the informed consent process.

Q16-C, HIV is reportable, and this patient has had the opportunity to discuss the matter with her husband. Physicians have a duty to report, if not done by the patient. Innocents victims and the public must be protected.

Q17-B Testing for HIV, as for any other medical procedure should be done only with the informed consent of the patient. The physician's role in the care of this patient is support, education, about her treatment options.

Q17-C, The Family's wishes can override a donor card.

Q18-D There is no good consensus on this currently. The only clear principle is that of non-abandonment. The physician should continue an ongoing therapeutic relationship and guide patient with information about his HIV disease and issues of addiction.

Q19-A This patient is exercising her right of decision making, autonomy. A Patient has the right to refuse life prolonging measures.

Q20-D uphold the health proxy.

Q21-B Dialysis is the procedure of choice to prolong life without intubation.

Q22-C The patient may proceed to surgery, without reversing DNR status.

Q24-B The competence of patient to give an ethically valid informed consent is doubtful. You should contact the primary investigator to discuss his participation in the trial. A surrogate who can give consent for participation is an option if it is patient's best interests.

Q25-A Futility is used inaccurately in many situations that appear undesirable. For this patient, treating pneumonia with antibiotics stands a reasonable chance of success. The patient's quality of life, though low, is still acceptable.

Q26-A Organ donation is a voluntary act. No one and no court of law has jurisdiction

Q27-C The Family's wishes can override a donor card.

Q28-D Elder abuse is common, and you have the right to report the abuse despite the objections of the patient. Although the legal requirements are not identical in all states, the ethical requirement of physicians to report abuse is clear and uncompromising.

Q29-D In cases of homicidal or suicidal ideation, the practitioner has a moral and legal obligation to inform potential victims and the proper authorities.

Q30- B The patient has autonomy over her own body.

Q31-E Physicians cannot revoke a driver's license. If any inconsistencies are noted, the matter should be discussed with the patient and he/she should be informed of the likelihood of danger.

Q32-B Physicians have the responsibility to protect patients from other impaired physicians. A physician is also responsible to help impaired colleagues by identifying sources for help.

Q33-C Signs of impairment at work may be absences, erratic behavior, mood swings, conflict with colleagues, and heavy drinking at functions. Impaired physicians may appear disheveled and disengaged. Clinical performance changes are signs of advanced impairment. Physicians may be hesitant to report a colleague of suspected impairment, to protect them, or fear the consequences, yet every physician has a duty of protecting patients from an impaired physician. Physicians should report their concerns about colleagues to the hospital impaired physician program, or to the chief of the appropriate clinical service.

Q 34-C Reporting of physical abuse is mandatory.

Q35-C Social and professional online presences must be kept separate, and professional conduct must be echoed in both areas.

Q36-C Physicians are ethically and legally obligated to disclose medical errors to patients.

Q37-D Physicians are committed to providing care without any professional conflict. If the patient or their family have different views regarding delivery of appropriate care, ethics committee involvement will be of benefit

Q38- B Physicians are ethically and legally obligated to disclose medical errors to patients.

References

ABIM Foundation. American Board of Internal Medicine; ACP-ASIM Foundation. American College of Physicians-American Society of Internal Medicine; European Federation of Internal Medicine. Medical professionalism in the new millennium: a physician charter. Ann Intern Med. 2002 Feb 5;136(3):243-6. PMID: 11827500

Baldisseri MR. Impaired healthcare professional. Crit Care Med. 2007;35(2 Suppl):S106-S116. [PMID:17242598]. See PubMed

Gillick MR. Advance care planning. N Engl J Med. 2004;350(1):7-8. [PMID:14702421]. See PubMed

Jones JW, McCullough LB, Richman BW. Ethical nuances of combining romance with medical practice. J Vasc Surg. 2005;41(1):174-175. [PMID:15696065]. See PubMed

Murphy JG, Stee L, McEvoy MT, Oshiro J. Journal reporting of medical errors: the wisdom of Solomon, the bravery of Achilles, and the foolishness of Pan. Chest. 2007;131(3):890-896. [PMID:17356109]. See PubMed

Snyder L, Leffler C; Ethics and Human Rights Committee; American College of Physicians. Ethics Manual: fifth edition. Ann Intern Med. 2005;142(7):560-582. [PMID:15809467]. See PubMed

Terry PB. Informed consent in clinical medicine. Chest. 2007;131(2): 563-568. [PMID:17296662]. See PubMed

Tonelli MR. Conflict of interest in clinical practice. Chest. 2007; 132(2):664-670. [PMID:17699138]. See PubMed

Farnan JM, Snyder Sulmasy L, Worster BK, Chaudhry HJ, Rhyne JA, Arora VM; American College of Physicians Ethics, Professionalism and Human Rights Committee; American College of Physicians Council of Associates; Federation of State Medical Boards Special Committee on Ethics and Professionalism*. Online medical professionalism: patient and public relationships: policy statement from the American College of Physicians and the Federation of State Medical Boards. Ann Intern Med. 2013 Apr 16;158(8):620-7. PMID: 23579867

Jonsen AR, Siegler M, Winslade WJ. Clinical Ethics: A Practical Approach to Ethical Decisions in Clinical Medicine. 5th ed. New York: McGraw-Hill; 2002.

Murphy JG, McEvoy MT. Revealing medical errors to your patients. Chest. 2008 May;133(5):1064-5. PMID: 18460511

Snyder L; American College of Physicians Ethics, Professionalism, and Human Rights Committee. American College of Physicians Ethics Manual: sixth edition. Ann Intern Med. 2012 Jan 3;156(1 Pt 2):73-104. PMID: 22213573

Clouser, K. Danner. 1975. Medical ethics: some uses, abuses, and limitations. New England Journal of Medicine 293: 384–387.

Weston, Anthony. 1997. A Practical Companion to Ethics. New York: Oxford University

Aulisio, Mark P., Arnold, Robert M., and Stuart J., Youngner. (eds.) 2003. Ethics Consultation: From Theory to Practice. Baltimore, MD: Johns Hopkins University Press.

Baker, Robert. 2013. Before Bioethics: A History of American Medical Ethics from the Colonial Period to the Bioethics Revolution. New York: Oxford University Press.

Jonsen, Albert R. 1998. The Birth of Bioethics. New York: Oxford University Press.

Pence, Gregory E. 2004. Classic Cases in Medical Ethics. Fourth edition. New York: McGraw-Hill.

Rothman, David J. 1992. Strangers at the Bedside: A History of How Law and Bioethics Transformed Medical Decision Making. NewYork: Basic Books.

Engelhardt, H. Tristram, Jr. 1996. The Foundations of Bioethics. Second edition. New York: Oxford University Press.

De Ville, Kenneth. 1994. "What does the law say?" law, ethics, and medical decision making. Western Journal of Medicine 160:478–480.

Hall, Mark A., Ellman, Ira M., and Orentlicher, David. 2011. Health Care Law and Ethics in a Nutshell. St. Paul, MN: West Publishing Company.

Liang, Bryan A. 2000. Health Law & Policy: A Survival Guide to Medicolegal Issues for Practitioners. Boston, MA: Butterworth-Heinemann.

McCrary, S. Van, Swanson, Jeffrey W., Perkins, Henry S., et al. 1992. Treatment decisions for terminally ill patients: physicians' legal defensiveness and knowledge of medical law. Law Medicine and Health Care 20: 364–376.

Macklin, Ruth. 1998. Ethical relativism in a multicultural society. Kennedy Institute of Ethics Journal 8: 1–22.

Council on Scientific Affairs, American Medical Association. 1993. Confidential health services for adolescents. JAMA 269:1420–1424.

Moskop, John C., Marco, Catherine A., Larkin, Gregory Luke, et al. 2005. From Hippocrates to HIPAA: privacy and confidentiality in emergency medicine – part I: conceptual, moral, and legal foundations. Annals of Emergency Medicine 45: 53–59.

Freedman, Benjamin. 1993. Offering truth: one ethical approach to the uninformed cancer patient. Archives of Internal Medicine 153:572–57

Grisso, Thomas and Appelbaum, Paul S. 1998. Assessing Competence to Consent to Treatment. New York: Oxford University Press: 31–60.

Moskop, John C. 2006. Informed consent and refusal of treatment: challenges for emergency physicians. Emergency Medicine Clinics of North America 24: 605–618.

Wicclair, Mark R. 1991. Patient decision-making capacity and risk. Bioethics 5: 91–104.

Berger, Jeffrey T., DeRenzo, Evan G., and Schwartz, Jack. 2008. Surrogate decision making: reconciling ethical theory and clinical practice. Annals of Internal Medicine 149: 48–53.

Pope, Thaddeus Mason. 2013. Making medical decisions for patients without surrogates. New England Journal of Medicine 369:1976–1977.

Committee on Ethics, American College of Obstetricians and Gynecologists. 2005. ACOG Committee opinion no. 321: maternal decision making, ethics, and the law. Obstetrics and Gynecology 106: 1127–1137.

Strong, Carson. 1987. Ethical conflicts between mother and fetus in obstetrics. Clinics in Perinatology 14: 313–328

King, Nancy M.P. and Moskop, John C. 2012. Advance care planning and end-of-life decision-making. In Hester, D. Micah and Schonfeld, Toby (eds.) 2012. Guidance for Healthcare Ethics Committees. Cambridge: Cambridge University Press: 80–87.

Moskop, John C. 2004. Improving care at the end of life: how advance care planning can help. Palliative and Supportive Care 2: 191–197

Von Gunten, Charles F., Ferris, Frank D., and Emanuel, Linda L. 2000. Ensuring competency in end-of-life care: communication and relational skills. JAMA 284: 3051–3057.

Council on Ethical and Judicial Affairs, American Medical Association. 1999. Medical futility in end-of-life care. JAMA 281: 937–941

Schneiderman, Lawrence J., Jecker, Nancy S., and Jonsen, Albert R. 1990. Medical futility: its meaning and ethical implications. Annals of Internal Medicine 112: 949–954.

Truog, Robert D., Brett, Allan S., and Frader, Joel. 1992. The trouble with futility. New England Journal of Medicine 326: 1560–1564.

Foley, Kathleen and Hendin, Herbert (eds.) 2002. The Case against Assisted Suicide: For the Right to End-of-Life Care. Baltimre, MD: Johns Hopkins University Press.

Rachels, James. 1975. Active and passive euthanasia. New England Journal of Medicine 292: 78–80.

Beecher, Henry K. 1966. Ethics and clinical research. New England Journal of Medicine 274: 1354–1360.

Levine, Robert J. 1988. Ethics and Regulation of Clinical Research. Second edition. New Haven, CT: Yale University Press.

Collins, Francis S. 2010. The Language of Life: DNA and the Revolution in Personalized Medicine. New York: HarperCollins Publishers

Veatch, Robert M. and Ross, Lainie Friedman. 2015. Transplantation Ethics. Second edition. Washington, DC: Georgetown University Press.